.

Season of Shadow

Season of Shadow

Chronicle of an Unwed Pregnancy

Jane and Amy Hudson

STANDARD PUBLISHING

Cincinnati, Ohio   29-03143

Scripture quotations are from the *New American Standard Bible,* © 1960, 1962, 1963, 1968, 1971, 1972, 1973, 1975, 1977, and are used by permission.

All of the people in this account are real, but Jane and Amy Hudson are pseudonyms, as are all other names throughout the book.

Library of Congress Cataloging-in-Publication Data

Hudson, Jane.
  Season of shadow.

  Summary: In their diary entries, a mother and daughter detail the pregnancy of the unmarried daughter.
  1. Teenage mothers—United States—Case studies.
  2. Unmarried mothers—United States—Case studies.
  3. Mothers and daughters—United States—Case studies.
  4. Family—United States—Religious life—Case studies.
[1. Unmarried mothers. 2. Pregnancy, 3. Mothers and daughters] I. Hudson, Amy. II. Title.
HQ759.64.H83   1989   306.874′3   89-4515
ISBN 0-87403-579-1

*"He who dwells
in the shelter of the Most High
will abide in the shadow
of the Almighty."
Psalm 91:1*

Contents

Preface

The pregnancy of our unwed daughter was a traumatic experience for our family. But through tragedy and pain, God brought a blessing and a strengthening to us.

During the process my daughter and I kept journals, writing down our thoughts and feelings as the months went by. By expressing the pain, the frustration, and the bewilderment of the situation, we hoped we could better understand what was happening, clarify our thinking, and be able to share this experience in an intimate, meaningful way as mother and daughter.

We share our journals in this public way, hoping that our experience can provide encouragement, comfort, and clarification to those who find themselves in the same situation. But every person and situation is different; we do not presume to know what is best for you or your loved one. The only advice we could give would be this: Explore all the options and depend upon God to guide you.

February

Two missed periods. What does it mean? I have always been somewhat irregular, but not like this. Is this why I've been getting sick these last few weeks? Could it really be happening to me?

Everyone is worried about me. They all think it is my ulcer flaring up. That could be it, couldn't it? But my ulcer has never caused me to vomit before. I have gained some weight too. That is unusual for me. I usually can eat and eat and never gain a pound. Maybe my metabolism is beginning to change. But my breasts are tender too. How can I explain that?

I am exhausted. I don't have the energy to do homework; I just want to sleep. I am too tired to get up and go to classes. My roommates only seem to see me when I am asleep on the couch. I am probably just sick with the flu.

Who am I trying to kid? I know what's wrong. I don't need a diagnosis. It's all the natural process of things. I have every symptom. I can't ignore it any longer. I am pregnant. Paul came back over Christmas break. Why did I agree to see him?

Why is this happening now? I am loving college. I love all my friends. I have grown so much. I am so much closer to the Lord. I have just begun to date Bryan, a wonderful guy. We get along so well; I can't remember ever being so comfortable around a guy. I feel as if I have known him for years. Am I going to have to give up this relationship?

I have to talk to someone. But who will understand?

I have told Heather, my roommate. She was shocked and wanted to know who and when; then, "Amy, do you know for sure?"

"No, but I have all the symptoms."

Then she hugged me and gave me her support. I will always love her for that.

I bought a home pregnancy test, followed the instructions. Waiting for the results, I thought over my evening with Bryan last night.

He knew something was wrong; I was so distant. I wasn't sure I should tell him, not knowing what he would think. But I need his support. His friendship has come to mean so much to me.

"What's wrong?" he asked for probably the tenth time.

"I'm not sure you really want to know. Bryan, I think I may be pregnant."

He was concerned and asked how I was feeling. I told him I was scared. He said he loved me anyway and then just held me close as I cried. He asked me about my relationship with the Lord.

"I feel so unworthy of His love. I have put Him through so much. This is bound to be the last straw. I don't know how He could still be there after what I have done."

Bryan reminded me that none of us deserves God's love, but that He does love us in spite of all we do. He asked me not to give up on the Lord but to give *in* to Him. And then we prayed.

I stop my remembering and look at the test results. Positive. The test is positive. My fears are confirmed. I should cry now, but I just feel numb. I can't cry, I can't speak; I feel nothing.

Yesterday I decided to call the university clinic. I shook inside as I told the receptionist my situation. She told me to come in and take a pregnancy test there, and then we would decide what to do. Heather said she will go with me. That's good; I need someone to lean on.

Then I decided to call Paul. My heart beat rapidly and my hands were trembling as I dialed his number. He sounded surprised to hear from me, and we just talked generally at first. Finally I said, "Wouldn't you like to know why I'm calling?"

"Yeah, sure."

"I think I'm pregnant."

"Oh, my God. Are you sure it's mine?"

"Yes, very sure."

"Have you been to a doctor?"

"No, I'm going tomorrow."

"Well, let me know the result."

Then we began to talk about what we would do if the result was positive. Surprisingly, he did not mention abortion. He explained that he knew I would not consider that an option. He suggested that I put the baby up for adoption. I agreed to think about that possibility. He was more supportive than I expected. We talked about our feelings.

After I hung up the phone, I decided to tell Melissa and Kerri—my other two roommates. When Kerri got home from work, Heather announced that we were going to have a "roomie" discussion. I then began to tell my "story." They expressed their love and support for me. I was able to rest a lot easier last night.

Today Heather and I decided to meet in the library after my last class and then go to the clinic. I thought of little else the rest of the day. I tried to sort out my feelings; they were so jumbled up. Thoughts were floating in and out of my mind. Thoughts of my family kept coming up. How will I tell my parents? They will be so disappointed. I never wanted to hurt them; I know this will hurt them terribly. I love them; why did I do this to them? I am especially worried about my dad. He has just been released from the hospital after having heart surgery. I prayed that this would not send him back to the hospital.

Heather and I drove to the clinic, talking about the "what if's." When we walked in and I looked around, all I could see was pregnant women and babies. Heather put her arm around me and said, "This is going to be you someday."

It was all over in a few minutes. Now we are to wait. I will call tomorrow for the results. The waiting is the worst!

I decided to skip classes today so I could call the clinic and then have some time to myself. Melissa and Heather sat next to me as I dialed the number. They were a bit excited. This whole experience is new to them, and they said they are looking forward to pampering me. I remember commenting that there was really no reason to call because I knew what the result would be. I was put on hold for what seemed like forever, but I finally got through; the lady looked through some papers and said the result was positive. I made an appointment to see a doctor. I hung up, and the three of us just sat there for a while, not quite knowing what to say.

I decided I would tell my brother first and started looking for him. He was about to leave the campus to go home, but he could see the urgency in my eyes and stopped to talk. I began to speak, but when I looked into his eyes I started choking on my words. He hugged me and let me cry. We talked for quite a while; actually, he talked and I cried. Each time I tried to speak, the words were muffled by my tears. I knew I was hurting him terribly and started to imagine the pain my parents would go through.

The rest of the day dragged on. I was in another world, it seemed. I ate lunch with Bryan, Heather, and Scott (her boyfriend) and discussed my situation a little. Being the people that they are, they tried to put some light into my darkness; that really helped. I went to work for a few hours but was sent home early. They could tell I was not feeling well. I decided I had to tell my parents tonight.

I started the half-hour drive home. I pulled into the familiar driveway, shaking more inside than out. Dad was upstairs, so I slowly climbed the stairs. He was surprised to see me; they were not expecting me home. I asked where Mom was and said that I needed to talk to them. He told me she was at choir practice at the church, and that I should go get her.

I was really uncomfortable as I pulled into the church parking lot, and thoughts of just forgetting it and going back to school crossed my mind. When I walked into the sanctuary where the choir was practicing, Mom spotted me and waved. I motioned for her to come. She gave me a hug and I told her I had to talk to her and Dad. She immediately gathered her things and came with me. A lump was forming in my throat as I drove, and I no longer knew what I was going to say once I got inside the house. All the words I had rehearsed disappeared.

The three of us sat around the kitchen counter. They were watching me anxiously.

"I made a mistake I will now have to pay for. I am pregnant. I'm sorry."

For a couple of minutes, neither said a word. As I watched the tears forming in my mother's eyes, my own began to fill. She was hurting for me and I couldn't bear to watch.

My dad's words were, "People make mistakes, Amy. We love you anyway." That was exactly what I needed to hear. He asked me what I wanted to do and what I was thinking.

"I'm not sure yet."

He asked about the boy and how it happened. I explained everything. He told me he wanted me to come home; he thinks it would be better for everyone if I were home instead of in the dormitory. Mom didn't say anything except, "Stay here tonight, Amy."

I told her I wanted to get back with my roommates

since I would have to leave the dorm soon. Dad told me to check into what I would need to do to move out by this weekend.

This weekend? He wants me home this weekend?! That is something I definitely am not willing to do. But I had no energy to fight tonight. So I left. I came back to an empty room. There was a note that Paul had called.

I called him back and told him about the result of the test and my talk with my parents. For about an hour we discussed what the next step should be. I do not know how to feel toward him. He keeps persisting that I should give the baby up and that he is not ready to be a father. Yet he was supportive of me, and I am beginning to think that maybe he really will help me through this.

This morning I explained to my roommates how the talk with my parents went, how they want me to move home but that I was going to try to fight that decision. After breakfast, I went to Dad's office to tell them (Mom is Dad's secretary) that I do not want to move home. I want to stay with my friends because I need their support at this time. But they didn't go for it, and I knew there was no point in arguing. They did say I could stay another week before coming home. So now I have time to say my good-byes.

The rest of this week has been devoted mainly to packing and saying good-bye. I told my closest friends my situation; everyone was great. A few didn't know quite how to react, but eventually they got used to the idea.

Some of my friends helped me move, which didn't take too long once we got started. I am sad about leaving, yet I know I will be around, so it won't be absolutely terrible. It seemed strange moving everything back into my room at home, but I know I have to make the best of it.

My emotions are really hard to understand. I am angry, upset, depressed, and scared—sometimes all at the same time. And every time I talk to Paul, we fight on the phone. He supposedly is trying to help, but I get furious with him. I try to explain what I am feeling, but it is too hard to explain, and he doesn't understand. I suppose I can't expect him to. He isn't going through any upheaval in his life, nor will he. I think that is why I am so angry. His life doesn't have to change like mine does. It just does not seem fair. The guy always gets the easy way out and, of course, most of them take it.

My relationship with Paul is what one might call strange. It began two years before at the home of a mutual friend. We did not exactly "meet." We acknowledged each other's presence in the same room, but we were not introduced nor did we speak. But the following night, he called, and we got acquainted over the phone. I was dating someone else at the time, but problems were arising, so when he asked me out I consented. I thought it might be just the right thing to find someone new.

After our date, I continued to date others because I did not want to make our relationship exclusive—I think I had an instinctive feeling that this match-up was not right. He doesn't live nearby, so it was not difficult to date others also.

One night I was visiting him at his friend's, where he stayed on weekends. He was going to be leaving in a few hours to go back home. We were sitting in the bedroom, listening to the stereo and talking. We kissed some, but when he began to go further physically than what I wanted, I tried to stop him. He did not like my saying no and pushing him away. He continued, and I said emphatically I did not want that and pushed him harder.

He responded angrily, "You are going to learn that you cannot turn me on and off like a light switch." He grabbed me harshly, pinned me down so that I could not move, and proceeded with his "plans." When it was over, he got up and said, "Now that wasn't so bad, was it?" Then he left the room. Shaking, I got dressed and left.

He continued to call me as if nothing had happened. But I could not pretend nothing had happened, and I wanted desperately to end our relationship. And yet there was a type of bond there, and I was extremely frightened of him. He knew where I lived; he knew where I worked. He knew where to find me if he wanted to hurt me again. I was so afraid of making him angry again; at the same time, I felt I was tied to him. This fear and the strange bond were the basis of our sporadic relationship from then on. I seldom saw him.

When he called over Christmas for a date, I consented because I was depressed, because I was still afraid of him, and because there was a connection with him. And when he wanted to be physically intimate again, I felt I had no choice or strength to combat him.

I can feel that now I am beginning to stand up to him—now that I'm pregnant, and he is being such a jerk about it. I was afraid of his reaction—afraid of his anger and what he might do to me. Yet I know that I have to be strong for my child's sake. I can't live in fear the rest of my life. And how can I ever forgive what he has done to me? Oh, God, help me be strong; erase this fear. Help me learn to forgive.

It can't be true. Maybe it is all a dream. Just a bad dream. When I wake up, all the pain, the hurt, and the sadness I feel right now will be gone. This could not be happening to us—not in our family. Oh, God, please let it all be a mistake!

Yes, there was a mistake. When Amy came to choir practice and said she had something to tell us, I was concerned and had a funny feeling in the pit of my stomach. At home in the kitchen, her whole body drooped; her eyes were filled with sadness; her voice was soft, as if fearful. "Mom, Dad, I've made a mistake—and now I'm going to have to pay for it. I'm pregnant. I'm sorry."

I was numb with pain. I was sure my heart was tearing into a thousand pieces. I wanted to scream but couldn't. I couldn't even get my breath or find any words to say. I felt a heaviness in my chest and stomach. I reached out to touch her because I knew what courage it took for her to tell us. I am sure she felt she would be shaming us, yet that aspect of the situation bothered me very little.

My main concern was the vast emotional and physical trauma that my beautiful and intelligent daughter will have to face. Her life will be marked and altered in a way that even I cannot fathom.

Sleepless nights. The sobbing, gasping, and groaning that came from Jack and me in the days and nights that followed as we hung onto each other in the privacy of our bedroom could not even begin to express our inner sadness and bewilderment.

Jack keeps saying, "We will get through this. We will face this. We will love and support her and help her get on with her life."

I cannot talk or think clearly. I can only feel—the pain, the hurt, the guilt. What did we do wrong? Jack blames his being gone so much during her growing-up years. I wonder if I did not talk with her enough about dating and her conduct with boys. Perhaps we were not strict enough. Perhaps we didn't watch over her activities and friends well enough. Or perhaps we were not the kind of Christian examples and models we should have been.

Now I am sleeping again, but I dream about babies. I dream all my daughters are pregnant. I dream I am pregnant. I live out in my dreams the pain and the heartache that I feel.

She was a freshman at a state university, doing well in her classes and making lots of friends—the right kind of friends. She was staying in the dormitory of a nearby Christian college. She had started dating a fine Christian young man. She had a very good job in the office of a small company, not too far from the university. She loved her work and her life. She seemed close to the Lord; she was attending a large church that had an active college group. She made friends there, participated in a discipleship group, and went to several Bible studies. She was so smart, so organized, so "together." She was so on top of things—how could this happen?

After she told us (that night in the kitchen), there was a long silence—at least it seemed long to us. Her father asked, "Who is the boy?" She told us his name. We didn't know him, had never met him, and couldn't even remember her saying much about him.

"Do you love him?"

"No, he's a jerk."

"Have you told him?"

"Yes. At first, he was real sorry and said maybe we ought to get married. But we both know it wouldn't work, because there is no love there. He said he would help financially and keep in touch. But unless I call him, we don't talk."

"Do his parents know?"

"No. They are divorced. He doesn't want them to know—especially not his dad."

She met him two years before through several other boys she had met at a county fair in a small town near us. She had dated several boys in that group but had never brought any of them home for us to meet. She was very independent then and wanted to be on her own, "running her own life," though still living at home. She did not feel that her parents had much to do with her life; we were "out of it" and did not understand—at least, that is the way I think she felt. She had her own car, and although we asked her not to go to boys' homes or be calling them all the time—she did anyway. She had a great need for the attention of young men.

Paul lives a few hundred miles away but came down on weekends to stay with his friends who lived near us. Amy told us that on one of those times in the bedroom of a friend's house, he forced himself on her in a brutal way. She decided then to stop seeing him and stop being with that group. It was hard for her to break away, but she did.

After seldom hearing from him for almost two years—on her Christmas vacation from the university—when she was feeling a bit depressed and lonely, he called her and asked her out. They went out for dinner and then back to the same house and the same bedroom. She said, "We got carried away. I'm really sorry. I was so hoping nothing would come of it."

I appreciated her honesty. She could have blamed the boy or said he had raped her again to save face— but she didn't.

Abortion was never an option for Amy. We all knew that. Amy and I both had gone through intensive training to be counselors for our church's pregnancy counseling center. She had written several papers in high school against abortion. She has firm convictions about the wrongness of it, for which I am very thankful.

But I can really understand how a girl could be tempted to use abortion—as a way out. It would certainly seem to solve some problems. Yet the sacredness of human life and a respect for the God we worship and the Christ we serve looms so strongly in front of us that abortion is no choice at all.

Amy and her father have pretty well decided that she will put the child up for adoption. She can get on with her life, make a couple very happy, and provide a complete family and home for her child. That decision seems logical and reasonable. But deep inside me, I feel a sadness. I have doubts about that course of action but have not expressed them to Amy. I feel very strongly that she has to make her own decision and do what is best for her.

She is so young and has her whole life ahead of her—a career (she wanted to own an accounting firm), marriage. I wanted her to have it all, and it would be so lovely and wonderful. But how can it be—now? She will have a child to support and care for. What are her chances for marriage now? How can she finish college and hold down a job that pays enough to support herself and a child? When will she have time to be with her child? Yes, it will indeed be easier and much more convenient to let a couple who cannot have children of their own raise and love her child—my first grandchild.

But I know what it feels like to have life growing within. I know what it feels like to hold a small, helpless human being, a person coming from your own flesh, through unspeakable pain and effort. I know the joy of seeing a child's first smile and feeling the first hug. I know the bond of love and possessiveness I feel for my own children—no power on earth could convince me to give up one who came from my flesh. Not even during the sleepless nights, the seeming spells of never-ending crying, the sicknesses, the tantrums, the heartaches. Watching children grow into real persons is my greatest source of happiness.

I wonder if Amy will feel that way too. I wonder if she will really be able to give up her begotten child. It would be an act of unselfishness, in a way. Yet when she feels movement and realizes the reality of life within her—I wonder. But the decision has to be hers, not mine.

March

We dreaded this in the worst way. But we knew we had to do it. Amy had already told her older brother, Mark. Now we had to tell her two younger sisters. We asked the girls to join us in the dining room; we told them we had to have a family conference. They came in quietly, seeming to sense that something serious was coming.

We told them that Amy had made a terrible mistake that would cause our whole family to make some ma-jor adjustments. We told them what had happened and how bad Amy feels. We explained that Amy will be moving out of the college dormitory and back into her room at home. We asked them not to tell their friends as yet. We want to have time to get our thoughts to-gether and decide whom we will tell at the outset. We told the girls we were going to try to be as supportive of Amy as we could be.

Jennifer, our youngest (ten), began crying uncontrol-lably, but Christi (fourteen) was very, very quiet. She went to her room and stayed there alone with the door closed for several hours. They both were frightened and wondering how it would affect us all.

Mark has been angry at Amy, saying she was really mixed up in her head to get in such a fix. I think he judges her more harshly than anyone else in the fam-ily—thinking of her as a "tramp." He talks often of how she has wrecked her life.

It is highly emotional for all of us, but we have be-gun to cling together more and even pray more specifi-cally about family matters. It is a dark time for us, a time when we go about our daily activities, but as if a shadow is hanging over us all.

I saw the doctor for the first time today, and I heard the baby's heartbeat. I was so excited, yet saddened because I felt I had no one to share it with. When I got home, I called Paul to tell him and share my excitement. He couldn't have cared less. Then I realized he isn't going to be around for me at all. In fact, he is going to do his best to put the whole thing out of his mind. This just adds to the anger I already feel toward him. I can't seem to forgive him.

My relationship with the Lord is strained. Because of me, of course. I have stayed away from church, because I felt that I did not belong there anymore. But realizing that Paul did not care made me feel extremely lonely. I had no one who could understand.

Finally, in seeming desperation, I decided to follow everyone's advice: I turned to God. When I felt no one else was there, He was. He put His arms around me, told me He loved me, and said, "Welcome home." He was still there for me, even though I have put Him through so much.

Amy, with the help of her friends from college, moved back home Saturday afternoon. How quickly her old room filled up again with her personal belongings! I felt sad, yet good and more secure about having her back under our roof.

The atmosphere was strained, for I didn't quite know what to say to her friends. Small talk seemed to be the best avenue. I was thankful that they did not rush off but stayed to eat with us. We spent an enjoyable afternoon swapping stories and "joking around."

But now her friends are gone—back to their own lives and pursuits. I'm sure Amy is wondering how often she will see them now and how her relationships will change. Her emotions are quite on edge, which is putting it mildly. It is a difficult time for all of us. There is a strange quietness in our usually bustling and noisy household.

I am trying to decide how to make things easier for all of us, but Jack was put back in the hospital today. He had two severe heart attacks in January. The doctors tried to get his heart stabilized before they took further diagnostic tests, but on a Sunday night he took a bad turn. The head cardiologist of the hospital stayed with Jack all that night, and I could tell he was very concerned, as was Jack. Jack was very emotional and tried to tell me amidst his pain what to do for the funeral. I have never been so afraid or felt so helpless in my life. I could only be with him a few minutes every hour; all I could do was hold his hand and watch his ashen face. He made it through the night, but the doctors decided he could not wait any longer and did surgery to open up his clogged arteries. He had a quick recovery and was doing well, although we knew that coronary arterial disease is progressive and *would always be with him in the months and years to come.*

We did not expect him to have recurring pain and problems so soon after the surgery, however. Thankfully, he does not have to have surgery again—just a regulation of his medication. He will be in the hospital for more than a week, testing various drugs.

As a result, I have not had much time to think of Amy or any home matters. I am keeping the office running in between visits to the hospital. The kids have been great, but they are worried. It is not easy for any of us. All other considerations have to be put aside while we concentrate on getting Jack to feel better.

Living at home has not been what I would call enjoyable. I've been bitter toward my parents for making me move away from my friends, and I've been
lonely and depressed. My emotions are mixed up,
and I don't know how to express them!

On top of coping with moving back under my parents' roof, I've had to face my pregnancy. I wanted
everyone to make it easy on me, but that hasn't happened.

Shortly after I moved back home, Dad was put
back in the hospital. Oh, Lord, what have I done?!
Not only have I let my parents down, but I have also
complicated my Dad's heart problems. Will this
nightmare ever end? If I hadn't messed up, Dad
would not be in the hospital again. Right?

Mom and I seem to be fighting a lot. I know she is
under a lot of stress with Dad in the hospital and
dealing with my pregnancy, but so am I. Mark and I
got into a fight about it.

"Amy, give Mom some slack. She's under a lot of
pressure."

"I know that, Mark, but so am I. I need some slack
too. I'm trying to understand her, but she needs to
try to understand me and my feelings too."

"You don't deserve any slack, and Mom does understand what you are going through. She's been
through it four times."

"No, Mark, she doesn't. She had a husband each
of those four times."

Then I broke into tears. I was so mad at him. He
wasn't even trying to understand. But he did stop to
think after my last statement, and put his arms
around me and apologized. Well, that's one step toward acceptance. Lord, give me the strength to cope.

April

I talked to the boy's mother today. Amy had told him that I wanted to. He asked her to stall me. He would tell his parents. I knew in my heart that he wouldn't.

I tried to call several times; a couple of times he answered, saying his mother was not home. I would hang up, wishing that I could tell him how I felt. He was a "rat," a manipulator, an aggressive macho male, sowing his wild oats (literally) in the bodies of many young girls (that is the way I pictured it). I wanted to tell him to stop being so selfish—to realize how hurtful he was being. But as he spoke, I knew that he was just a young college boy, and the probability of his listening to an angry mother was slim indeed.

But I hoped that if his mother knew, maybe it would make a difference. I had planned what I would say to her, but when she answered, I could hardly get my breath or get a word out. My face felt hot, I could feel my heart pounding in my ears, my mouth was dry. I almost hung up and thought, "I will try again tomorrow." Yet my desire to know more about this boy— who he is, what his family is like, what is going on in his life—was stronger than my desire to put this experience off another day. I had to talk to her.

I told her whose mother I was; she recognized Amy's name immediately as a friend of her son. "She used to call all the time," she said. I told her of Amy's situation and her son's part in it. I described what went on in her son's friend's house on the weekends when he came down to visit.

She said she was very sorry and that her son was very aggressive and popular with girls. She asked about Amy's plans. I told her that we were Christians and did not believe in abortion, so Amy was consider-

ing have the child adopted.

She talked of her own life—how she had divorced when her boys were young, raising them as a single parent, trying to see that they kept busy in worthwhile things so they would not get into trouble. Her younger son is bookish and a loner, but Paul, the older, is a roller-skating champion and quite gregarious. He is not working but going to a community college at present.

She said she is sorry about what happened and that they would do whatever they could to help. But then she talked about her financial problems, and I knew as she talked that she really does not intend to do any-thing—that she and her son will just forget it. Amy is in this alone. I gave her my phone number, but she has never called.

Why does the girl have to be the one to pay for the mistakes of two people? He can go on his way, probably impregnating a few more girls. And what is our responsibility as Christians? Make a fuss? Demand money? I am troubled and confused about this aspect. And not a little angry too—a whole lot angry. We have to endure this, while he and his family get off free.

Whom do you tell something like this? Do you tell everybody you know? Write special letters? Send out a news release? Or do you keep it quiet, hoping no one will notice?

We have not wanted to tell anyone. It is not that we feel particularly ashamed or guilty, but I think it is the fear of rejection, criticism, and being judged as "deficient Christians." We didn't know how our friends and acquaintances would react to the news. Would they continue to be our friends? Or would they say nice things to our face while gossiping behind our back?

Some of our friends, of course, have had similar traumas or disappointments in their families—so surely they should understand. Yet, it has been our experience that often they are the very people who are most judgmental and critical when other families have difficulties.

We decided to tell the staff at the office and a small group of friends at church. We will not send out a bulletin or a newsflash to our friends all over the country. We would tell only when it became necessary to do so.

The people at the office were very supportive and sympathetic. Those who have had similar experiences told us their stories and offered counsel and comfort. We felt surrounded by warmth and did not feel alone any longer.

Every Monday morning I meet with a group of women for Bible study and prayer in preparation for the weekly women's Bible study at our church—an organized women's group of which I am leader and co-teacher. During prayer time, I tearfully told of Amy's situation and how it was affecting our family. I asked for prayer, especially concerning decisions that would need to be made about the welfare of the child and what we should do about the father's lack of responsibility.

It was as if a dam burst forth—the women began sharing (also tearfully) about their own experiences. There were two women whose daughters had experienced the same thing. There was one woman who had given a child away several years ago and has regretted it ever since. On and on the stories went. There was much crying, hugging, and saying, "I know just how you feel" and "Things will be all right, although it doesn't look like it right now." Our meeting went an hour overtime, but in those moments we grew close in care for one another and in understanding.

That group has remained a constant source of comfort and encouragement to me. A great deal of discussion with this group about whether it would be best to put the child up for adoption or keep the child was an enormous help to me. It enabled me to think through those decisions so I could be more of an "informed" help to Amy. I thank God for these women, who opened up their arms and hearts to me at a time when I most needed it.

This whole issue of "whom to tell" and fearing reactions of friends and acquaintances has made me reevaluate my relationships. It makes me want to be the kind of friend who is supportive and loving no matter what the problem—extending God's grace as freely as He does—the kind of friend who is not critical or judgmental, leaving judgment to God. That kind of friend is what I need most at this time.

*All of our friends and relatives have been very sym-
pathetic and supportive. We were afraid to tell them;
I'm not sure why—we know such things happen often
in families these days. But, of course, we didn't expect
it to happen in our family. I guess our pride was hurt.
We have always been so proud of our children. They
are bright, well-liked, superachievers. It's hard to admit
to others their mistakes and failures—even hard to
admit to ourselves.*

*My parents came at Eastertime. I wanted to tell
them and planned to do so as I took them to the air-
port to return home. I didn't want to ruin their visit. Of
course, they wondered why Amy had moved back
home instead of staying in the dorm. And I'm sure
they noticed how she vomited every morning in the
bathroom. Amy complained a lot about a backache
and generally not feeling very well. So we talked about
the possibility of her having the flu. What a coward I
was!*

*As it turned out, Jack took my parents to the air-
port; he didn't want to tell them. He says we don't
need to tell our relatives in the Midwest unless Amy
decides to keep the baby.*

*But I knew I had to tell my parents. I could not keep
such a major happening in our lives from them. So I
telephoned them the next day. Dad answered. Mom
had gone out for a while. I told him the story and explained why I didn't tell them earlier. He was very understanding, though saddened. He said they loved us
and would be praying for us.*

*A few days later, Amy got a beautiful and touching
card from my mother.*

*My mother has called a few times and told me of
other family members who have gone through the*

same thing and how the young single mothers who decided to keep their children are doing. She has been an encouragement to us, and I can often feel the comfort and love across the miles.

I know that I need to go back to church. I can't handle this by myself. I need the support of fellow Christians if I am to succeed in putting my spiritual life back together. I already know about God's love, how He was still there after all the pain I had put Him through. His arms are open wide and He is ready to pour His love out on me if I am willing. I now understand the true meaning of the parable of the prodigal son. I was a "prodigal daughter"; I didn't really expect God to still be there, but I am so grateful that He was.

I've begun going back to church. I only put one foot in the door for a while; I wasn't sure whom I could trust. The more I go, the more comfortable I become. Only a few know about my pregnancy, and I still am not showing, so it is easy to hide. I can see the difference God is making in the youth group and I want to get involved once again. I need to be plugged in to a church family, and the more I pray about it, the more I feel the Lord's leading in that direction. But I also know that, for myself, I will have to tell the entire youth group about my pregnancy.

That thought is so scary. How will they react? Will they support me or reject me? I continue to pray about it, hoping that God will tell me I don't have to humiliate myself in that way. I know that I am all right with God and with my parents, but am I all right with myself? That is the question I am forced to answer. I know I have not yet truly forgiven myself, and I also know that I won't unless I confess my sin to everyone.

Tonight was the night. I knew that at this Bible study I had to confess. Before Steve, our youth pastor, began to teach, he told us to listen to the Lord during prayer time. So I asked God again, "Do I really have to go through this?" He told me that if I wanted to have peace within myself and if I wanted to be involved with this group, I would have to confess.

During the invitation time after the study, I stepped out and walked into the counseling room. Donna already knew about my pregnancy and had said she would go with me. We prayed together. I was shaking uncontrollably and again wasn't sure that I wanted to do this. But I had to; I knew God would give me the strength somehow.

When the group was finished singing, Donna walked up to the microphone, introduced me, and said I needed support and prayer. I looked out at the two hundred faces staring at me and spotted my sister. When I looked at her, I knew that she knew what I was going to say. She put her head into her hands. Tears filled my eyes and I began to speak.

"A couple of months ago, I found out that I am pregnant. I am four months along now, and I need your support and prayer."

Not knowing how the group was going to react, I went back to my seat. After Steve dismissed us, I stood up and was immediately surrounded. Everyone was offering support and reached out to me in love. I wasn't expecting so much acceptance from them. Because of some of my past experiences with these same young people, I expected to be rejected or judged. But they surprised me. How thankful I am! The changes that I thought had taken place in the youth group proved to be true. There is love there, and I know that I will be comforted, not isolated.

Thank You, Lord, for giving me the strength to confess my mistake. And thanks for giving everyone an understanding heart. I never could have said anything if You had not been by my side. Now I can begin the process of forgiving myself, for I no longer have anything to hide.

Well, I suppose Dad is right. I can't financially take care of a baby, go to school, and spend the time with my child that I would want to. I guess I shouldn't deprive the baby of the chance of having a father.

Heather told me about a couple who want to adopt. I gave her my work number to give them and they called. I agreed to meet with them after work on Monday. They sound like neat people, but I am scared about meeting them. But God will be with me.

They have been looking for a baby for three years. They are so ready; they even have a nursery fixed up. They have two names picked out. They would be wonderful parents, I feel sure.

Dad is thrilled that I liked them so much. Mom seems uneasy. I am wondering why. Does she not want me to have my baby adopted? But she has never said a word either way.

Something is tugging away inside of me. I don't understand why I feel restless. They are a wonderful couple; they deserve to have a baby. But should they have mine? Lord, please let me know what You have planned for me.

Today Heather told me what the couple said about me. They were very impressed and felt that I have a good head on my shoulders. They said they would love to have a daughter like me. I am so glad to hear that they liked me as well as I liked them. Maybe that is my answer.

This morning I felt my baby move. It was so exciting. This was real! I knew I was pregnant but a large part of me just couldn't believe it. I have a living person inside of *me*. Depending completely on *me*. I am a mother. I never thought I would feel this way. I never understood the concept of a mother/child bond until now. I never thought I would love this child so soon, so much. How am I going to be able to give up this child?

After classes were over, I went to Mom's office to tell her. She smiled and, as tears filled her eyes, she said, "It's amazing, isn't it, Amy?"

"Yes, Mom, it is."

"Amy, I just want to tell you that if you want this baby, I will do whatever I can to help you."

Immediately, I began to cry. Mom finally told me how she felt. In a way, I could hardly believe what I was hearing. Was there a way I could keep my child?

I had already told the couple they could have my child; yet right before we were to begin legal proceedings, I had second thoughts. Could I really give my child to someone else and be satisfied with the possibility that I might never see him or her again? Would I be able to live with myself? I am not sure. I want my baby, but is it the right thing to do? Lord, please show me Your will!

My parents and I have decided that I should go through some counseling to help me sort out my options. If I think them through thoroughly with an objective person guiding me, then I will be able to make a good decision. I will go to a Christian crisis pregnancy center in our area.

She felt the baby move. I will never forget the look on her face when she told me. Her eyes were wide, her face glowing; she almost laughed and squealed with amazement and joy. She held her hand on her enlarging abdomen and said, "I felt the baby move today, Mom. He's poking around in there. I'm beginning to love this baby."

I have trouble describing the way I felt as I listened to her—joy, yes ... awe ... some fear ... a tightening in my chest ... tears welled up in my eyes ... I couldn't get my breath and could barely respond to her. I mainly smiled. I guess the best way to say it is that I am overwhelmed with the thought that my child is going to have a child.

May

Amy amazes me. She is not depressed or gloomy. She is not down on herself. She has a positive, optimistic attitude. She loves life. She looks at her situation with a great deal of humor—her attitude is infectious. We are all able to deal with this reality with a brighter outlook because of her. If it were me, I would be very depressed and introspective. I would hide from others.

She keeps in touch with all of her Christian friends from church and school, goes out with them, has them over, and has a great time—quite silly and hilarious at times. I think she is dealing with everything in a very healthy way. I'm so proud of her. She has taught me how tough situations can be met.

She is bold in her witness of how the Lord is controlling her life and helping her face this difficulty. She seems to be always conscious of His presence. The joy she feels shows—even as the child within her is "showing" since she is getting larger and larger every day.

Of course, there is the possibility that she is not really facing up to reality, that she is making this be her time in the limelight as kind of a heroine, or that she is hiding her real hurt and self-incrimination. But I don't think so.

Jack was gone for the weekend, so I decided that we girls needed to get away. I reserved a hotel room at a nearby resort, and we drove down on a Saturday morning—Amy, her two sisters, and me.

We got into our room, unloaded our luggage, and went exploring. We had a good time, wandering from shop to shop, oohing and ahhing and giggling . . . lots of giggling. We watched a juggler present an exhibition and took lots of pictures. We watched the people and ate ice cream and these huge frankfurters.

We were laughing so hard at one point that Amy's sister said, "Be careful, Mom, you will have a heart attack."

"No, that would be your dad," I replied. "I would get a big hive." (I have had a case of hives since December.)

Amy said, "Well, I might have a cow."

I said, "No way, you're not big enough."

Her sister said, "But you haven't seen the father, Mom." We laughed until the tears came and everyone around us was staring.

We were all able to laugh and joke about Amy's pregnancy. A good sign, I think.

She wants to keep the baby. She says she knows it won't be easy. Kids her age are so idealistic. I have raised four kids—I know it won't be easy. There is no way she knows how truly difficult it is going to be. I ache for her. Yet I understand.

Her eyes brim with tears as she says, "I feel the baby moving; I am beginning to know the baby. I love this baby. There is no way I can give him up."

Her dad is aghast, even though I warned him that she might be feeling this way. We had a discussion around the dining room table.

"As a father, I must tell you that I don't think it will be best for the baby's welfare. There must be a tight bonding with the mother during the child's first two years of life—how can you provide that, and work, and get your degree?"

"I think I have lots of friends who would help me. I am planning to have three thousand dollars saved by the end of the summer. I could put off going to college for a while or take night classes. And Mom said she would help take care of the baby."

"Your mother would have to quit work, then. We would not be able to get you a new car as we had planned. Your car has over eighty thousand miles on it and may not last much longer.

"If you are not a full-time student, you will not be included on our group insurance policy after you turn nineteen—which means you will need to plan on close to two hundred dollars a month for medical insurance for you and the child. The baby will require many trips to the pediatrician; there may be pharmacy costs. There will be furniture and supplies needed for the baby—a nursery, food, and clothing. You can live here at home, but it will be extremely difficult for you to

meet these costs with your present salary, even working full-time.

"And we don't feel we should make the other kids suffer. Mark will have college expenses; Christi will be entering high school with all the extra expenses that will bring. We can cut out vacations and our luxuries, but even at that, our living expenses are enormous. It will be especially difficult if your mother has to quit work.

"You need to think about what will be for your child's good—not only what you feel emotionally."

Harsh reality, isn't it?

She was so looking forward to tonight. She had arranged for her father and me, herself, and a Christian young fellow she especially likes (and had dated some before she discovered her pregnancy) to go to a dinner theater. She wanted us to meet him; he was interested in music as a career, so she thought a musical and a dinner would be enjoyable for all.

She looked so beautiful. She took special care to look nice. It was obvious that she likes this young man very much; her excitement about our meeting him was unusual.

The evening was everything she had hoped for. Conversation was lively; the musical was entertaining. She looked so soft and feminine; her eyes sparkled; she laughed often. I sensed that they both genuinely liked each other—yet I felt that Amy's feelings were more like love.

I ached for her. I knew (in a partial way) the pain she will feel as the months go on when her love is not returned. It would be a rare person who would want to get seriously involved with a pregnant girl, or even a single mother and child. I can picture in my mind the deep hurt that is coming to my daughter in the months, maybe even years, ahead. I cried inside and felt quite low by the time we got home.

The feeling was still with me when I went to the worship service this morning. As we were praying and singing, the tears started flowing and I could not stop them. Worship that morning completely disarmed me. My defenses, my walls, came down—tumbling down—in waves. The feeling that I have to be strong ... I have to have courage and hope ... that I must hold myself tight so I don't fall apart—in worship I released it all. I felt relief, but I also felt pain.

Things were becoming clearer ... and reality loomed large with crystal clarity. The Holy Spirit was working within me and revealing to me the truth. He was washing away the clouds of confusion in a very rapid and organized way. He was revealing to me my weaknesses, my wrong thinking, my wrong motives—it was as if I stood naked before God, with no more reserves, only full dependence on Him.

All these many weeks I have been rationalizing, thinking logically, making lists—and yet I was totally befuddled and overwhelmed with it all. But in that worship service, the truly significant loomed large, and the insignificant took its rightful place. I was cleansed. I was humbled. I made promises. I felt comforted. And I began to hope again. I know now that even in my weaknesses, I can stand. And even if and when I fall, He will be there!

June

I told Mom that I am definitely thinking about keeping my baby. I told her I will continue to work part-time and go to school if she can baby-sit. She says she will, and we have been brainstorming ways to work it out.

Mom told my dad that I am considering this option, so he said we needed to have a long, serious discussion about it.

"Amy, how do you plan on keeping the baby?"

"I thought I could work in the afternoon, be home in the morning, and go to school at night. Mom could baby-sit when I can't be with the baby."

He then began to lay out all the financial responsibilities. I had already thought of most of them and hoped that my parents would help me out. But the way Dad was talking, I am not so sure. He even said he isn't sure that Mom will be able to quit her full-time job because of our dependence on her salary.

We talked about what is best for the baby. Dad is determined that he or she would be better off with adoptive parents. He thinks that the child will have identity problems otherwise. He also thinks I will not be able to date or get married, that no young man would want a ready-made family. But I know that is not necessarily so, and besides, dating is not that important to me anymore.

I tried to explain to Dad how I feel about my baby and how I would feel about giving my baby to others. I could not be sure how my child would be treated or if the marriage would be intact as the years went on. The discussion ended with me in tears and Dad terribly upset. He does not understand and wants me to do what he wants; he does not seem open to any other way but his.

We went to the mall for a day of shopping. Amy needed some clothes, and I thought this would be a good chance for us to talk. We really enjoyed trying on clothes and getting each other's opinion on how we looked. Amy wanted to get some cool summer casuals that would be big enough now but also wearable after the baby is born.

She was so pretty . . . but getting larger. She had to try on sizes that she would have never thought she would be wearing—she's always been a size 3; now it's size 9 or 10. But we picked out nice accessories to dress her outfits up . . . she really looked cute.

The mall had a television star from the "General Hospital" soap appearing soon on the center-court stage, so I saved our seats and held the packages while Amy went to get us some sandwiches. We ate as we waited and we talked.

First, we listed the advantages to the child if she kept him or her:

1. The baby would be with its natural mother and grandparents.

2. The baby would be in a loving home atmosphere.

3. There would be no feeling of rejection later, except from the standpoint of the father.

4. There would not be the extreme emotional hurt for Amy to have to give up her child.

Then we talked about the disadvantages:

1. The child would have no father figure. Amy says her male friends will help, but I told her she can't count on that. They have their own lives to lead and will not be available very often.

2. The financial burden. She said, "I will nurse the baby; we will go to rummage sales; perhaps someone will give me a shower; I will go to school maybe even through the summers, get my degree and then get a good job."

3. *The restriction of freedom.* She will not be able to participate fully in church or school activities; she will always have to think of someone else. She said, "I am well aware of that. I am willing to forego my freedom in order to fulfill my responsibility. So there will be no new car, no vacations, and probably no dates for a while—I don't care much about those things anymore. I have a new view of life."

Just then we saw this beautiful baby in a stroller not far from us. He was laughing and trying to get out of the stroller. He was a fat little thing in a Pamper and a red-striped knit shirt; he had only a wisp of hair, big blue eyes, and a grin wider than his face.

We watched him, laughed, and said, "How cute!" Yes, Amy notices babies now as never before. And talks about how sweet and cute they are.

I hope she is not idealizing the role of mother and thinking of the baby as a little doll to hold and play with. I hope she realizes that they cry and make messes.

I talked to her about those aspects, and she said she has been warned by another girl who kept her baby of the realities of raising a child. She wanted me to know clearly that she is not wearing rose-colored glasses. She says she doesn't feel she will be a nervous, worrying mother or let a crying, fussy baby bother her. That is not her temperament pattern, I agree, but who knows? No one knows for sure.

Jack has worked over our budget backwards and forwards, cutting out every "extra" he could—even considering asking Mark to pay more of his college expenses than he is already. Without my income, our life-style will be greatly changed.

And considering the long term, if Amy works and goes to college, it will be a long time before she gets her degree and a good-paying job—one that could support her and the child adequately. Plus the fact that she would not be able to be with her child very much.

We took Amy out to dinner one night to discuss the financial aspect again and made clear to her the not-too-pleasant realities of her decision.

She was saddened. She did not realize the financial aspect would be so rough, and she had been counting on my taking care of the baby (more than I realized) when she couldn't. Her secure feeling that her baby would be in a good environment and have good care was severely shaken by this discussion.

What is the right decision? Is God the only one who knows? I woke up this morning picturing Amy at home with the baby, juggling her college classes, nursing the baby, and trying to be a "together" person. And someday having to answer the question, "Where is my father?" I ached for her.

I pictured the baby in a home with adoptive parents who were able to provide the time and financial security that a child needs. I pictured them being very happy and complete now, despite not being able to have a child of their own. But . . . I also could hear them face the question, "Why did my mother give me away?"

Amy was getting ready for work. I stood at the door of her room and shared with her the two pictures that had crossed my mind and asked her if she had pictures like that.

"Yes, Mom. All the time." She was crying now. We sat on the floor, held each other, and cried. "I wish I knew the right thing to do. I've prayed about it so often, but it doesn't do any good. I don't get any answers."

We prayed together then, asking for God's wisdom and guidance, recognizing that He knows and cares how we are agonizing.

She told me that evening that she wished God would send down a telegram giving her step-by-step instructions of what she should do. We laughed. Then she told me about her friend Rose (from work), who has an illegitimate son and no contact with the child's father. She told Amy there was nothing easy about it, but it could be done. She lived with her parents for a long time and is now married. She said her son has had no identity crisis and no desire to see his father.

He is in junior high and loves his stepfather very much.

Amy took encouragement from her friend's experience. I thought to myself, "Yes, but Amy, it is not always that way." Then I also thought, "Could this be the beginning of some type of guidance from God?"

Please, Lord, I need to feel Your peace, Your direction, and Your comfort. Help me to be at peace with whatever decision she makes.

Mom, Dad, and I went out for dinner. As we started to eat, Dad brought up the topic of discussion—my baby. He asked me what I had decided. I told him once again that I want to keep my baby. He then began to lay out our family's financial situation. I soon discovered that we can't afford to have Mom quit her full-time job to work part-time and take care of the baby while I go to school. We need her salary. I thought, "But I want my baby. There has to be a way! Why are the doors closing on me now when they had seemed to be so open and I felt everything was so right? Is God trying to tell me something, or is Satan trying to maneuver his way into the situation to make me doubt? I am so confused."

When we got home, I went to my room, sat on the bed, and cried. I don't want to give up my baby, but now it looks as if I will have to. Dad is telling me that what I want is impossible. But is it? Oh, Lord, help me!

As I was sitting on the bed, I picked up a book on adoption that someone had given me and began to read. I thought maybe this *is* God's way of telling me that I should give my child to a couple. Hardly able to see because of the tears, I wrote a letter to my child:

My darling child,

I love you so much! I can't even begin to find a way to express it fully. I've made many decisions concerning you. I seem to have just been going back and forth since the day I was told that I was carrying you. You see, all I truly want is the best for you. I want to do what will make you the happiest.

My first decision concerning you was to carry you

to full term. It's so easy these days to just get an abortion. But I could never do that to you. You had a right to live, and you deserve to have a wonderful life. I wanted you to *live* above all else!

I then had to decide whether to try to raise you myself or to give you to a couple who could give you so much more than I could. My decision had thus become much more difficult. Where *you* would be most happy was what was truly in question.

I began to think through what I wanted to give to you so that you could have what you deserve. I began to try to see how I could support you on my own. I began to lean on the Lord for support. I knew He would know what was best for you and where you would be the happiest.

I then began to realize that all I had to offer you was love. And a great deal of it, I might add. I could not possibly support you the way I would want to. So I decided to look into adoption. Quickly, I found a couple that I felt would give you love, support, and a "family."

But shortly before we were about to proceed with those plans (I was four months pregnant), I began to have second thoughts. I began to have less and less inner peace with the decision. And though I had never ceased praying since day one, my prayers became more intense. I wanted to do God's will, for I knew He had your best interest in mind. You also began to move inside me. I truly felt the sense of motherhood. My bond to you was and is so natural. I never really knew or could even imagine how it would feel, but my love for you began to grow stronger and stronger.

How could I possibly give you up with all this love

I felt inside? I did not know. But how could I support you? I did not know. I continued praying as our lives moved on, and I talked to my parents about keeping you and raising you myself. So plans were made. I would quit work so I could finish school. My mom, your grandmother, would quit her full-time job so she could work part-time and baby-sit while I attended classes. As soon as I graduated and got a good job, I would move out on my own.

I felt that doors were opening, and I felt such a joy and peace with my decision; I felt that this was what God wanted. But sometimes when we, as people, plan things, thinking that it is in God's will because there is an open door, He says, "No, that is not what I meant."

You see, my dear, God always knows what is best for us. He can see further down the road than we can. And He has specific plans for all of us. We stray from that plan many times, and sometimes we become confused in what we think His plans are.

If I am to be totally honest with myself, I can only say that I had begun to think more about my feelings and wants than your happiness, well-being, and needs. But now I see that you deserve both a mother and a father who love each other, who will love you, and will give you the life you deserve. You will be happier in the long run with them than you would be with me. It has been hard for me to realize that, but I hope someday you will understand that I did it all for you.

I want to explain to you about your birth father. We dated for about two years off and on, but we never got along. Why we continued to see each other, I don't know. Each time we did, it was at a lonely time for both of us. One of those times was when you were conceived. We were far from being in love; I will always regret that you were not conceived in love. You deserve so much more than that. Neither of us planned on having a child, and he did not want to face the responsibility.

Please don't misunderstand. Because you were not created in a loving relationship does not mean you were and are not deeply loved. For you are loved, with a love that is too deep for expression with mere words. It is an eternal love. For as long as you live, you are loved greatly by me, your mother.

I will forever carry a part of you with me, for you are a part of me. No person or thing could ever break the bond we have. I will miss you greatly, yet I pray that you will understand that what I did was purely out of love for you.

If love was all that was in question, the decision would have been so easy. If love was all you needed to have the life you deserve, I would have kept you without hesitation. For I do love you. But, honey, I realized that love alone does not get you everything I want you to have and what you deserve. I know that someday you will understand.

Love, your mother

When I finished, I said this prayer: "Lord, I am having a hard time with this. I want to keep and raise my child, but the doors seem to be closing. I am not sure what to make of it. Are you telling me that adoption is what I should do? I want to do what You want for me. Please allow the couple that I first picked to still want my baby. They are the only people I would feel at all comfortable with. And Lord, I will need You to help me. I don't know how I will be able to do this." Then I cried myself to sleep.

The next morning I woke up in a terrible mood. I was very depressed. Mom came in and asked how I was feeling after our talk the night before. I pointed to the letter on my desk, and as she picked it up, the tears welled up in my eyes again. I sat in my bed and cried as she read what I had written, and as she read, she started crying too. When she finished, she sat down beside me and put her arm around me.

"That is a beautiful letter, Amy. Is that how you really feel?"

"I think so, Mom. I can't force everyone else to sacrifice because of me. I want my child to have the best. I *think* God may be telling me that adoption is best."

I broke into tears again, with my mother's arms enveloping me. The two of us cried together for what seemed like hours. Finally she spoke, "Amy, I guess you should start looking for a couple then." I nodded.

"But keep your mind open and keep praying about it. OK?" Again I nodded. That is something I am certainly going to do. I have to keep asking till the very end. Maybe there is a *slight* chance I can keep my baby.

July

Tonight was my first meeting with Carol, the counselor at the pregnancy crisis center. My parents are on vacation, so they don't know I am starting my sessions. Carol asked me questions about myself and my family. She then asked about the baby's father and about my relationship to him. She gave me a workbook to fill out, and we will go over my answers when we meet next time.

I have met with Carol three times. We talk about the questions in the workbook and my answers. We have explored the options of adoption and of keeping the baby. I realize that I have no peace about adoption; I have begun to feel strongly that this would not be best for me or the child. When I make the right decision, I believe the Lord will give me a peace about it.

Tonight I called Paul to tell him that I have changed my mind. I was shaking as I dialed his number, for I have not talked to him in months. We began with small talk; then I said, "I called to tell you that I am planning to keep my baby."

"You're kidding, right?"

"No, I am serious. I just wanted you to know that you will not be getting any adoption papers to sign."

"Why are you doing this?"

"Because I want this baby; I love him or her even though I don't love the father."

"Now what? I don't want this to interfere with my life. I want nothing to do with it."

"Fine. I just wanted you to know. Good-bye."

So that was it. I could force him to support the child. I could take him to court and drag him through the dirt. And I could probably win. But then, in later years, he might want to see his child. I don't want him in my life or around my baby. He has not wanted to help, and I know that he would never be a good father. His involvement would only cause problems. No, I will let him go and do it without him. What he did was unfair, but I am not about to let him get involved years later down the road. If he doesn't care now, he never will. I know I will never hear from him again.

Mom found out that I don't have to put his name on the birth certificate. That way there will be no danger of his taking my baby away from me.

When my parents got back from their trip, I told Mom what I have decided. "Mom, I am not at peace with the option of adoption, and I know I could never give my child away."

Mom told Dad, and I know he is not too happy with my decision. But he said that if that is what I want, we will try to work it out. He says that perhaps I should quit work and concentrate on going to school to get my degree. That way I would get out sooner and be able to support myself and my child. My parents would have to support me and my baby fully until then.

Everything seems to be fitting into place. God is opening so many doors. Is this what He has had in mind?

Jack is the type of man who sees things only one way and makes quick decisions. He decided as soon as Amy told us of her pregnancy that she would give her child up for adoption and the whole episode would be forgotten. He made it clear that there was no room for discussion.

I felt it was much more complicated than that and that there were other options that needed to be investigated before a decision could be made. I wanted Amy to do what was right for her and the child—what was right in God's eyes—not what I wanted or what her father wanted. Because I was very unsure of what was God's will in the matter, I have prayed constantly and asked God to give us all insight and guidance. I have been determined not to manipulate or try to sway Amy or Jack in any way. "Let God do the guiding" has been my philosophy.

Jack has been the realistic and practical one, thinking about the financial strain and the problems that keeping the baby would entail. Amy and I have been thinking emotionally, concerned about the child's future feeling of being rejected by his father and mother. Why have the child go through that unless it is absolutely necessary? We also know that we could provide the child with a loving and caring environment.

As time goes on and discussion continues, Jack has begun to mellow out. He is beginning to see that there are other options and that Amy's emotional state and desires need to be considered. This process has certainly not been comfortable for him—his health is still a vital consideration, and he has always had such a huge sense of the financial responsibility he carries for his family. But God is working and guiding.

I admire my husband for his many good qualities

and for how well he balances out my thinking and attitudes. But I admire him most of all at this time for his willingness to change and grow, even though his basic temperament does not make it easy for him to do so. His consistent study of the Word and his prayer life enable him to mature beyond his temperament and personality traits.

The final decision has not yet been made in any of our minds, but I can see that his mind and heart are opening up.

Tonight we attended Parent's Night at the hospital. Their philosophy and procedure of childbirth were explained. They showed us the labor and delivery room (same room) and explained what to expect when labor begins.

Husbands and their pregnant wives filled the room— I wondered how Amy felt when they talked about the husband being the coach in the labor room, and seeing all the other couples there.

I felt sad and a bit dismayed. So much has changed since I had my last child! Natural childbirth and breastfeeding were not encouraged when I was having babies. And now I am to be Amy's coach to help her through labor and the birth. Will I be able to do it? She will only be in the hospital for twenty-four hours if all goes well. Then she will go home ... Then it hit me full force—this is real. My daughter really is going to have a baby! And I will be an active participant in the process. Another baby is actually going to be in our home after all these years! What changes and adjustments will need to take place!

Next week we will start going to the natural childbirth classes taught by a nurse. I'm scared.

Tonight was my first childbirth class. Mom went also because she plans to be my coach. I was nervous as we walked into the room. As the teacher called out the names, I surveyed the other "students." I was the youngest one there; most of the others were husband and wife; there was one other mother/daughter team. I thought I would feel really out of place, but I didn't. After all, I had something in common with most of the women there. We were all going to have babies and were there to learn about the birthing process.

Each class has been very interesting. I learned a lot about my body and what would be happening to it as I gave birth. The birth of a child is an absolute miracle, I am beginning to realize. A miracle that only God could have devised, I am convinced. How anyone could not see God's part in it all is beyond my comprehension.

I am so glad I decided to have Mom be my coach. We are learning together and having a great time besides! It has given us time to spend together and to talk. Our relationship is changing from mother/daughter to friends. I am now seeing her as a wonderful friend. I never thought that this pregnancy would draw my mother and me closer together, but I am so thankful it did. I know that the Lord is the reason for that.

Thank You, Lord, for bringing good into what I thought of as a lifelong tragedy.

August

Preparation for Childbirth Classes:
I have had four children but never attended a preparation for childbirth class. I went to it initially to be with Amy, to be a comfort and support to her. The teacher could tell her what she needed to know—then I wouldn't have to.

But I found myself being absolutely fascinated with what was being taught. I am astounded at all that I did not know. I had never fully realized how carefully God planned our bodies for the purpose of childbearing and nurturing. The nurse who taught the class emphasized all the physical aspects that are for the baby's protection while being formed in the uterus and during labor, how labor is a natural process, and how important physical and emotional health are in the delivery of a healthy baby.

Even though I have been through the experience of childbirth and read books about it, I never realized the magnitude of what God did for women when He designed us for giving birth. I was asleep through most of the births of my children and was not fully aware of how awesome and God-related it all is. I am no longer so frightened about helping Amy through it. I feel extremely privileged to be a part of the experience in this way. Few mothers will get this type of opportunity. I appreciate God's creative hand even more now and appreciate the privilege of sharing this experience so fully with my daughter. I am so excited and delighted. I feel like telling the whole world about it!

Last night I came down to the beach, where my family has been staying for a week. But today only Mom, my sister Jennifer, and I are here.

We lay on the beach for a couple of hours this morning. Mom and I began to talk about the baby again. But the conversation took a different turn.

"Amy, I showed your letter to the baby to your dad. I hope that was OK."

"Oh, sure, it was. What did he say?"

"He said he thinks there might be a way you can keep the baby. He doesn't want you to think it is impossible."

"What? Why has he changed his mind?"

"I suppose his heart is changing somewhat." Then she told me about a conversation Dad had recently with a girl whose sister had a child out of wedlock and how her father had opened his heart to take the child into the family. She showed him a side that he had never looked at before.

My dad changing his mind! That is something I never expected! Is God answering my prayers? Is this God's will in my decision? Could it be that God is making the way clear for me to keep my baby?

I began to tell Mom all that the Lord had laid upon my heart recently. I have been reading *The Pursuit of Holiness*. This statement hit me: "One of Satan's chief weapons is discouragement." To me that means that when we feel we are following God's will, Satan will step in and throw something at us to make us believe we are not.

The Lord also showed me these verses: "But if God so arrays the grass in the field, which is alive today and tomorrow is thrown into the furnace, how much more will He clothe you, O men of little faith!

And do not seek what you shall eat and what you shall drink, and do not keep worrying. For all these things the nations of the world eagerly seek, but your Father knows that you need these things" (Luke 12:28-30).

Those verses tell me that the Lord will provide the means if I just turn the problem over to Him. After reading these verses, I felt so strongly that God wanted me to keep this child.

I told Mom, "I am going to make my plans for keeping the baby. If I happen to be off base in my interpretation of what God is telling me, I know He will reveal it to me in time."

I also explained to Mom about my prayer concerning the couple I had previously chosen—the day after I prayed that prayer, I heard that they had found another baby. I think God is telling me what He wants for me. I have made my decision.

I met a guy at church and we have begun to date. We get along wonderfully and are determined to keep our relationship focused on Christ. Neither of us is really sure why God put us together at this time, but we know for sure He did. I have been able to share all my thoughts and feelings with Jon, something I have not experienced in a relationship before. He is very special indeed.

Jon and I talked tonight about what things will be like after the baby is born. We know it will be different, for we will have less time to ourselves. I will have a big responsibility, and one that will take a great deal of my time. I did assure him that I would make time for our relationship because he means a lot to me. I asked him if he would be able to handle the change, and he said he isn't sure but that he will try. We decided to take one day at a time, and we will both try to handle the changes as they come.

Jon talks to the baby in my tummy all the time. He is interested in my child and seems to love him already. That means a lot to me. His desire to be involved in my child's life is special to me. He is special to be willing to go through this with me when the child is not biologically his. So far he has planned to stick by me now and after the baby is born. But I will accept it if he discovers he can't handle it. I hope he can, but I will understand if it happens to go the other way.

Jon told me that he was praying the other day and asked God if he is going to be able to handle it after the baby is born. He said that God seemed to tell him that if he trusted in Him, he will be able to. That helped so much, to know that Jon is taking our relationship before the Lord.

Since Amy has definitely decided to keep her child, we are needing to get the house ready for a new little person. We decided to move Amy upstairs so she could have a room, the baby could have a room, and Amy would have her own bathroom. That means the other two girls would need to move downstairs and Mark would move to the room we had built in the garage (for the foster daughter we had with us for two years). He is seldom here anyway and said it would be fine. While we were moving furniture, I decided it would be a good time to paint all the rooms and get the whole house spic and span.

I approached Mark with the idea of the project, and he agreed to help me. I didn't want Jack doing heavy work or being overly stressed out, so we did most of the work while he was gone on a trip.

I prepared the rooms and did the detail work, while Mark handled the roller. It turned out to be a great time for Mark and me to talk about life, about his future, his goals, and about Amy's situation. He was the first person in the family whom Amy told that she was pregnant, and he was also the most judgmental about it. After she told him, he talked for several weeks about her "looseness" and stupidity in getting into this predicament.

Mark has been upset that Jack and I have "caved in" (as he put it) to Amy's desire to keep the baby. He felt it was just going to cause more problems and that I would end up taking care of the baby. Why couldn't she just give it up for adoption and go on with her life? Why were we supporting her in this decision and agreeing to financially support her and the baby while she goes back to college? This could take years!

I told him that we felt Amy needed to be the one to

make the decision because it was definitely traumatic and would affect her the rest of her life. "We could not force her to do something against her convictions without causing great harm to her as a person. We know that anything could happen when the baby finally arrives on the scene—I am well aware of what I might be letting myself in for. But Amy has never been irresponsible and has never gone back on her goals or her promises. She simply made a mistake at this time in her life. I am glad she feels so responsible for her mistake and that she loves her child as much as she does. Yes, she may think things are going to be rosy when they won't be—they will be difficult, but she will adjust and so will all of us.

"Isn't that what families are for? To support and help one another when wrong turns and mistakes are made or when times are hard? To do all we can to make life livable for each other? To cooperate with each other and not take advantage? That is why God put us in the family—so we could share joys and sorrows, so we could be proud of great achievements and help mend the hurts and mistakes, so we could be the proper environment for maturing persons toward the likeness of Christ—which means extending grace as well as discipline.

"We intend to support and love Amy and be the group that holds her accountable for her actions. We want her to grow and mature and be able to get past this time in her life with as few scars as possible. How much sadder it would be if she had no one to support and comfort her in a decision that she feels God has guided her toward. Yes, our family and situation will be changed, but God is in it.

"Besides, this situation has made us all act more like

a cohesive family than we have in a long time. Just look how we are working together to get the nursery ready! Your sisters are planning to baby-sit and are thinking about ways to decorate the nursery."

Mark was silent for a while. Then he said, "You know, Mom, I think you are right. That's what families are for."

My son and I felt quite close in that moment, and that conversation will be forever etched in our memories. We both matured somewhat, and I felt God was smiling. Before that moment, I had not verbalized why we were handling the situation in this manner. It was as if a moment of insight enriched us both, even while we were spotted with paint and perspiration.

Not only did Daddy buy me a new car for my birthday, but he also bought the baby a beautiful cradle! I was so surprised, yet so happy! Is he finally coming to accept this child? Oh, Lord, You are changing his heart so he will be able to love this child. Mom kept telling me that he would change, but I just didn't see how. Jon and I put the cradle together (since Dad hates putting things together); it was so neat to work side by side getting ready for the baby. It seemed to bring us closer together. Everything seems to be working out. God has done wonders for me and my life.

September

Dad has just told me something that I never thought I would hear from him. Lately he has just been full of wonderful surprises!

"Amy, I just wanted to tell you that I think you made a mature decision about this baby."

Tears began to fill my eyes as I realized that he had come to full acceptance of my decision and my child. Thank You, Lord, for now I know I made the right decision. I know now that my entire family is happy about the child that is to be added to this family.

Today was my baby shower. A few of my closest friends got together to throw me a beautiful shower—a day I will always remember. All of us had a wonderful time playing games, eating, and I enjoyed opening all the gifts. The time is getting closer, and it seems so much more real now. I am getting more excited as each day goes by and as I look at the little clothes and rattles. It is hard to believe that I will be a mother in less than a month!

Today was my last day at work. I knew when I left the house in the morning that it was going to be difficult. I loved working there and loved the people I worked with. I had even built up friendships with some of the customers. I didn't want to leave these friendships behind. The day began like any other, but to me it wasn't the same. People called to say good-bye, and each time it seemed to get more difficult.

I went to lunch with a friend, and when I returned, I realized that half the day was over. When I walked back into the office, there were a few presents on my desk from some of the people I worked with. As I opened the baby gifts, tears filled my eyes but I blinked them back. I did not want to cry. I continued all day saying good-bye, so that in a way I was ready to go home at the end of the day.

But it was as hard as I had feared. The boss's wife came in to say good-bye and give me a gift. She and her husband had already done so much for me since I had started working there; they did not need to do anymore. And I couldn't hold back the tears anymore—especially when I saw what they had given me, a baby swing! Now each time I put my child in it, I will remember the wonderful people I worked for and how they had become such special friends. I was crying openly as I hugged everyone. They all wished me the best and asked me to keep in touch. Inside, I knew I could never forget these special people.

Tonight Jon and I broke up. He was beginning to have a hard time since the big day is coming so soon. The reality of the changes that were about to occur set in, and he was not able to handle it. He was beginning to feel boxed in and somewhat scared of what it all could mean. I am terribly hurt, yet I understand. It would be hard for any guy to handle the fact that his girl friend is about to have someone else's child. I have told myself that if this happened, I would accept it, but now I am having a hard time doing so. I need him more than I realized, and now I am due in a little over a week. How could he do this now?

He said he doesn't want to lose me, and I thought for sure that we could hang in there and work it out, for our relationship seemed so strong. I was sure we could endure this. I told him that we should not just give up. I told him I do not want to lose what we had and asked if we could try until the baby comes, and then we would know what changes there would be and go from there. But even after I made my little speech, he said he felt it would be better if we were just friends and did not date.

Friends? How can I just be his friend? I am in love with him! But I do need his friendship. I will have to try to do it his way. I didn't cry at first; I wanted to be strong for him. I knew he needed me to be at that moment. I needed to show him that I will be OK, yet I wasn't sure I would be. But if I wanted him to be happy, I knew I would have to let him go. Of course, it is never as simple as it sounds. It will take a long time. I have been crying ever since he left, and I will probably cry myself to sleep tonight.

I have gone through a whole range of emotions this last week. The breakup with Jon is only part of it. I am also excited about the baby coming and so full of love for my child. I can't wait to see the wonder that I have been carrying around for the last nine months. I also feel fear. Will I be a good mother? Will anyone ever want to get close to me again? Will I lose my friends? Will I really be able to raise a child and go to college at the same time? Will the delivery be hard? Will I be able to endure the pain that I have heard so many stories about? Will my child love me as much as I already love him or her?

Suddenly I know that God is with me and that I will be OK. The day I have been waiting for and preparing for is coming soon, and everything will be fine.

October

It was 3:15 A.M. I was awakened by a sharp pain in my abdomen. It only lasted a few seconds, but ten minutes later there was another one. Was I going into labor? I wasn't sure, but I began to time the contractions anyway. They were irregular for a while. But when I moved around, the pain would not go away. After a half hour passed, they began to be five minutes apart and became regular. Now I was more sure that this was it.

At four-thirty Dad came upstairs to see what was wrong. He could hear me moving around, since their bedroom is right below mine.

"Amy, are you OK?"

"Dad, I think I'm in labor. The contractions have been five minutes apart for forty minutes now."

"Well, I'll wake Mom up."

A few minutes later, Mom was in my room, asking how strong the contractions felt. I told her they did not feel too strong yet.

"Well, let's try to get some more sleep. Keep timing them and see if they get stronger."

I agreed and lay down once again. They were still five minutes apart, and after a while they were a great deal stronger. Finally at five-thirty I decided to wake Mom up again. I now knew that this was it and began to get excited. I had been waiting for this day and it was finally here. As I was walking down the stairs, Mom was coming up.

"The pains are getting stronger and are still five minutes apart, Mom."

"OK, we had better start getting ready to go."

I went back into my room and packed my bag. I then made my bed and brought everything downstairs. Christi and Jennifer were both awake by now too. All of us were getting excited. A new family member was about to be added. Everyone took a shower and got dressed. Christi and Jennifer were allowed to skip school and go to the hospital. Mom called the hospital and told them I was coming in. Then the five of us sat in the living room, held hands, and prayed.

At seven we were in the car headed for the hospital. It was rush hour so we were stuck in traffic. But I was concentrating on my breathing and didn't notice the traffic much. We arrived at the hospital at eight. The room wasn't quite ready, so we waited in the waiting room for a while. Mom and I were allowed in the labor/delivery room a little after nine. I was so excited! This was it! The day was here, and my life was about to change in the most wonderful way!

The midwife checked me and said I was halfway there and that it would not be long. I got comfortable, trying to relax by listening to my tape of classical guitar music. Mom gave me ice, timed my pains, and massaged me. I was given something to help me relax. Very soon after that, the pains became very intense and two minutes or so apart. Then I felt like I needed to push.

Mom called the nurse, and things started happening. All the equipment was brought in—even the warmed bed for the baby. At 11:03 A.M., my little boy was born! The midwife laid him on my stomach. As I looked down on this miracle from God, who had been a part of me for so many months, the tears of joy began to flow—and they were not only my tears—my Mom and the nurse were also shedding a few and smiling at the same time.

Eric Matthew, you have already brought so much

joy to my life, and I can't wait to watch you continue
to grow. How beautiful you are! I love you, Eric, with
all my heart. And I thank God that He blessed me
with you; what a wonderful blessing you are!

The rest of the family was allowed in the room for
a few minutes and each took turns holding him.
They all seemed so proud and yet shy, not knowing
exactly what to say, but all looking in wonder at the
miracle.

I was actually calm. I was afraid I would be overly excited and not be of much help to Amy, but I was calm—even as we were on the freeway in the worst traffic snarl I have ever been in. I knew we had time, and Amy was doing her special breathing technique very well. Jack had stayed behind at the house to call Mark and would be following us soon.

When we arrived at the hospital, I realized that the nurse who had taught the childbirth classes was on duty. What an unexpected bonus! Amy and I both sighed with relief. She was glad to see us and excited that she would participate in this event with us.

As soon as Amy was put in bed, things began happening rapidly. Her pains intensified, the midwife said she was well along, and I could only think about playing her tape of relaxing music, rubbing her arms, feeding her ice chips, and encouraging her to do her breathing during the pains.

Then the moment arrived! What satisfaction and overwhelming excitement as we struggled to bring this baby into the world! Amy did it like a pro! It was an incredible experience. When we saw the head emerge, followed by the body of the not-so-little boy—the feeling and joy were indescribable. He was perfectly formed and crying—yet looking around in wonder at his new world. We were all surprised at how big he was, because Amy had never gotten large.

He was here! How excited we all were as we took turns holding him. We were all moved soon after delivery to a rooming-in room. The baby stayed with us the whole time. The family could come and go as they wished. Many of Amy's friends came by to visit and see the baby. We were all proudly showing him off. No one was more proud or excited than the men in the family. Mark kept saying, "Look at my nephew—the most perfect baby I have ever seen." And Jack kept talking to Eric in long lectures about life.

At one point, when there was a bit of quiet, I turned to Jack and asked, "Could you give him up to another family?"

He got this incredible look on his face—like a light had gone on—and answered, "You know, I think it would be impossible. He is a part of us."

Yes, Eric Matthew Hudson is a part of us. All of our lives will be altered from this moment on. We are in this together.

Epilogue I

When I was a sophomore in high school, I began to pull away from God and the church. I felt pressured by my parents to go to church and to live up to their ideals and values. I guess I decided to rebel against all that and find out who I was as a person on my own. But instead of concentrating on finding out who I was or what I wanted, I got caught up in my rebellion. I was having lots of fun and becoming very self-centered. I even forgot why I was rebelling; I was rebelling just for the sake of rebelling.

I did not trust in God to guide me or to shape my future. I took the first things that came along, giving no thought to God. I was taken in by the very first guy I dated. I really thought I had fallen in love; we were planning on being married, even though our parents kept saying we were much too young to even talk about it. I figured that since marriage was in our plans, it would be OK to give myself to him in every way. As soon as I gave myself to him physically, our whole relationship centered around sex. Finally the pressure for sex got so intense (while the love and caring got sidetracked) that I had to end the relationship to have any peace within myself—something was very wrong. The breakup was difficult; neither of us handled it well.

But that type of relationship so early in my dating life left its mark. As time went on, it seemed that a lot of my self-worth was tied up in sexual expression with a guy. I should never have depended on a relationship so fully to secure my self-image. I should have trusted in God's love for me to realize my value and worth.

While I was wandering outside of God's will, I also lacked good judgment about people. I became careless in my choice of friends and whom I dated. I hung out with non-Christians and became involved in their way of life. I adopted their values and continued to push aside all that I had been taught at home and church. I gave in easily to peer pressure in every area, except drugs. Thank goodness I had enough strength and sense to stay out of that! Though I did not always enjoy what I said yes to, it always gave me a sense of fitting in, belonging, and being of value. I didn't get that feeling in any other way—that was because God was no longer an active ingredient in my life.

These attitudes and actions I wish I could change, but I do not regret having my child. He is the beautiful that God brought out of my ugliness. When I first found out that I was pregnant, I was devastated and thought it was the end of the world. I had already gone through so much; how could I possibly make it through this? It was hard for me to see what was ahead. I felt like I was going to break apart.

Many people quoted Romans 8:28 to me: "And we know that God causes all things to work together for good to those who love God, to those who are called according to His purpose." But each time I heard it, I could not see what good God could make out of this. Yet He showed me how. He taught me a lot about His character and what it means to have a relationship with Him. He taught me to be dependent on Him and to give Him my all. When I finally learned that, I knew He would take care of me and never let me fall. I learned what His love really is. He still loved me, although I had hurt Him terribly. He was there to put the pieces back together. He forgave me with no questions asked and was determined to use me for His work. He let me know that I have a friend in Him.

God taught me and He blessed me. I now have a beautiful son, one whom I could never give away or exchange for anything in the world. I am so thankful that I have him. I truly could not imagine not having him now. Each time I look at him, I thank the Lord for giving Eric Matthew to me.

My family and I are closer now than ever before, and I thank the Lord for the friendships He allowed me to find inside my own family. The Lord has also given me a new type of ministry. After going through this, I can help other girls who go through the same thing.

For me, the Lord showed me that keeping my son was the best. That may not always be the best for someone else. Trusting in the Lord and accepting His guidance is the main thing.

Yes, bad things happen to good people, to Christian families. As our children were growing up, Jack and I were very aware of their developmental stages and needs. We consistently sought to provide them with a loving, stable, Christian environment—filled with laughter, work, and good times. We made it a point to be good examples and to teach Christian values and attitudes. Christ was usually our focus (we got off on other things—like material aspects—at times), and church was certainly our main activity and environment outside the home. Even though others said it would happen, we really didn't believe that any of our children would become rebellious teenagers who messed up their lives. But it happened.

This was a crushing blow to us. I felt for a while that though we had tried hard, we were just not good enough as parents. I wondered if maybe our home had not been as stable and loving as we had always thought. I wondered if our personal Christianity was really valid; had it been real all these years?

The hurt and the pain were setting in, causing me to doubt myself and the life we had built together as a family. Desolation was gripping me. My husband was seriously ill; my unwed daughter was expecting a child—I felt so helpless. I wanted to make everything right, but knew that I couldn't. I was sinking into a murky, shadowy zone—wondering if or when the light would return.

Time passed. The world did not stop. Our friends were still our friends. We were all pulling together as a family, supporting one another—even beginning to laugh again. Our faith was still there; God was still showing His love to us.

I learned that after our children reach a certain age

(different for different people), they will experiment and seek independence; they will seek to find out who they are and what values and attitudes they want to keep as well as which ones they want to discard. And much to our chagrin as parents, they will make mis-takes along the way (no matter what we say or do)—some mistakes that will alter the course of their lives. This is all a part of their maturing process, and the part that we as parents have little control over (unless we are harsh dictators). This is the time we need to rest in constant prayer and realize that God loves our children even more than we do. I came to realize that if I failed as a parent in any way, it was in the area of prayer—I didn't pray enough.

A joyful and satisfying by-product of this experience is that my daughter and I have become much closer and gotten to know each other better. I discovered that she is a truly nice and good person who is compas-sionate (almost too much so) toward others. If she has a fault, it is that she is naive and too trusting. I am very proud of her and count myself very fortunate to have such a daughter—but even more important, I am very blessed that she has become one of my best friends.

My daughter has also taught me a valuable lesson about how to face adversity—not to retreat and hide in shame, but to face it squarely with head held high, with a positive cheerful view, and a hopeful outlook. Include your friends in your pain; don't shut them out, and, most of all, be honest.

I also developed a more intimate relationship with my God. I learned what His faithfulness and steadfast-ness mean to everyday life. He cleared away the shadows and the pain; He took care of us financially (through friends and family all the baby's needs for the nursery, clothing, and supplies have been met); He brought good out of a bad situation. He waited patiently when we failed to focus on Him; He comforted us with His Word; He gave us peace through prayer. He made clear the right path. He has blessed us in a beautiful way. I cannot praise the Lord enough for what He has done in us as individuals and as a family!

I have also learned what an overwhelming joy there is in being a grandparent to the most precious child on earth. The love I feel for him is so huge and growing each day. When he smiles and responds to me, pockets of joy burst within me. I miss him terribly when I'm not with him. There is a powerful bond there; it is hard to describe, but different from the parent/child relationship. The added blessing of having my grandchild live with us and seeing the love that we are all extending to that child warms me all over.

I am sure that troubled times will come, but I am also sure that God will be there.

Epilogue II

Five months after Eric's birth

A youth group in a neighboring community was having a series of lessons on sex and dating; they asked Amy and me to participate on a panel to share our experiences and give counsel to the young people and their parents who would attend. There were two other women on the panel—one who had had two abortions, and one who had given her child up for adoption.

I prepared my talk—a simple sharing of my feelings, what I would advise young girls, and what I would have done differently as a parent. I did not take time to think about who would be there or the various reactions that might occur. My main concern was that I get through my portion of the program without crying buckets of tears. Amy and I both knew that it would be difficult because we had not spoken publicly about this difficult time in our lives. We decided to bring the baby with us as a live "object lesson."

I was totally unprepared for what happened. First, in the process of explaining my feelings, I got off on a tangent about the boy who had raped my daughter on a date and then came back into her life, expecting an intimate sexual relationship, and then refused to take any responsibility for the results of his actions. I talked very strongly to the boys in the group about their demands of a girl in a dating relationship and was surprised at the anger and frustration that I felt and was expressing for the first time—in a public way and completely unplanned. I admitted to the group that I suddenly realized that my anger toward the boy had not been resolved.

My second shock was the reaction of the group in the question-and-answer session after the discussion. It became quite obvious to me that the group all

139

favored the avenue of adoption and thought we were incredibly stupid and selfish to decide to keep the child.

I wondered how they could possibly think that when they could see the beautiful and happy baby in the room. How could they think that Amy was selfish when she changed her whole life around for that child? Her focus was now completely on him and his welfare. The girl on the panel who had given her child up for adoption was dating, going to college, and continuing her life as if nothing had happened. She was free of all responsibilities toward her child and could live her life as she pleased. How was she being more unselfish and righteous? Was it that her child would be better off with two parents? What guarantees do we have of that in this society filled with divorce and child abuse?

At least Amy knows that her child is loved and well cared for. She will never have to explain the rejection of both parents to her child. Her child will always be sure that he was loved and wanted and that his mother fulfilled her responsibilities to him, regardless of the inconvenience to her own life.

We were not given the opportunity to defend our actions or decisions, but perhaps someday we can. And yet, the important thing is that we know we did what was best for us and the child. God has blessed us abundantly in that decision.

Epilogue III

One year after Eric's birth

My grandson is now one year old. To have been able to have such an integral part in the earliest days of his life has been the source of great joy to me and to the rest of the family. I have heard others say that grandparenting is the best part of life. Now I can say it truly is. The special relationship is different from that of parent and child. I have tried to determine what makes it so different and so very wonderful, but I have not come to any conclusions as yet.

I am sure you are wondering what problems we have encountered since we made the decision to keep this child and incorporate him into our family. I can honestly say there have been problems—but only a few; the joys have been multitudinous.

He is a healthy, extremely intelligent, beautiful child. (This is a grandmother talking, but everyone agrees.) He has had no major illnesses or traumas. He has been walking for several months; he is talking and feeding himself. He loves dogs. He loves to rough-house and cuddle. He is very inquisitive (that's putting it mildly) and so affectionate. His face lights up when he sees us; there is no doubt that he loves each of us.

Amy has taken full responsibility for him and truly loves motherhood. It is hard for her to be apart from him even for a short while. She has endured the sleep-less nights, the trips to the doctor, the days of teething and fussiness, and his propensity to explore. She has combined working, going to college, and motherhood. She has been so tired some weeks that she slept most of the weekend. I was relieved when she decided to quit work. Though the money was helpful, she needed to be with her son and have more time to rest and study.

A major problem was finding the right baby-sitter. I

never had to do that when raising my children, so I had no concept of how difficult that can be. I truthfully hated the idea of her leaving him with someone else all day long. I am now able to watch him the two days that she goes to classes. How much better we all feel about that arrangement! We know what is happening with him; we don't have to wonder. And he is thriving! He is so much more content to be in his own home and with those he knows best rather than being up-rooted each day.

Amy is able to devote more time to him and her studies, which has proven to be the best thing. She made almost all A's (one B) this semester.

Jack is a doting grandfather and loves to play with Eric. He still gives him long lectures about the meaning of life and takes him outside with him when he works on the cars or in the yard. He is always very con-scious of providing the right environment for him—plays "good" music (as Jack calls it) for him instead of what the teenagers play. Eric loves to sit with Grandpa in the big recliner and "read stories."

Our other children have responded so well to the disruption in their lives. They all love Eric and fight about who gets to hold him or play with him next. In the mornings when we are all getting ready for the day, he makes the rounds of our rooms (padding around in his pajamas)—getting a hug and a kiss from each, looking into a certain drawer or getting some-thing off a certain shelf to hold, and saying the same things to each, "What's ya doin'?" and "What's this?" This has become a morning ritual.

He welcomes us all with a special look or touch when we come home and has certain activities that he enjoys with each of us. He knows Grandma is always

146

ready to feed him, so they enjoy snacks together and watching movies on the VCR (like "Winnie the Pooh" and "Lady and the Tramp"). He reads stories with Grandpa; he expects Mark to chase him or throw him in the air; he loves to go through Christi's drawers; and he expects Jennifer to play with him on the floor with his toys whenever he wants to—and she usually does. And, of course, no one else can comfort him or console him when he is hurting or sick but his mother.

We are delighted that a special young man has come into Amy's life. He is filling a need in her life as well as Eric's. They are planning marriage in the future, but are wisely not rushing into it—for which we are very thankful. There is a lot of growing up to do for both of them before they attempt marriage. We continually pray that God will guide in this matter. We know that He cares about Amy and her son even more than we do.

Finances have been tight but not unmanageable. We don't go out or entertain as often, but we have not missed that aspect of our lives as much as we thought we might. We have other things to fill up the spaces. Our needs have been met. We feel no lack. We have learned to economize and do without.

Our situation at this time is good. I have a hard time thinking that my life could be more fulfilling than it is right now. God has worked wonders in us. I thank God every day for what He has done for us and in us—as well as for what He has in store for us. Things seemed so dark and hopeless at one time; then the light peeked through the shadows. Now we are enjoying the full and amazing light of God's grace and presence in our lives.

Epilogue IV

Fourteen months after Eric's birth

It has been fourteen months since Eric was born. The time has flown by, and I have seen him grow into a wonderful and happy little boy. He has filled my life with so much love and joy that I could not describe it adequately. Being responsible for helping him grow is an experience I would not trade for anything. I do not regret in any way my decision to keep my child—even though it has not been easy.

When Eric was nearly four months old, I returned to my classes at the university. It was so difficult that for a while I thought it might be impossible to be both mother and student, but as it turned out my grades and retention of what I learned were better. I think it was because my life had been refocused; I now had a better reason for going to school. I now wanted to improve myself so I would have more to give my son. The most difficult part was leaving him with a baby-sitter, but she was a personal friend with a young child of her own, so that helped.

I decided to start working again in June. I wanted to help my parents financially by at least working during the summer (no classes) while my sisters could baby-sit. I went out on a lot of interviews and was getting discouraged, but then God provided a job for me just five minutes from our house. When school started again in September, I talked my boss into letting me work three days a week so I could go to classes the other two days. My parents tried to talk me out of trying to work and go to college also, but I was determined to show them that I could do it.

At first things went OK. My baby-sitter lived just a few houses down the street, so I could come home and have lunch with Eric on my break. But when college was in full swing and the assignments grew, I found myself studying a lot and not sleeping much. I caught colds often and was not having nearly enough time with my child. By the time I got home from work or classes, there was only an hour to spend with Eric before he went to bed. Then I would study till midnight and get up at four to study again.

After two months my baby-sitter quit because of personal problems. To think about having to check out new baby-sitters just seemed overwhelming at the time. I was not enjoying working that much, so I decided to spend my time studying and mothering, and I quit my job.

My social life was greatly reduced after Eric was born; I had expected that, but there were a few surprises along the way too. While I was pregnant, the church youth group was extremely supportive, but after Eric was born, I felt all alone as far as friends were concerned. At first many brought gifts and visited, but when the newness wore off, very few called or were interested in how things were going. And then when we *were* together, they gave all their attention to Eric and didn't seem to have much to say to me.

It really bothered me at first, but I began to realize that I was a different person. Our situations in life were quite different, and I couldn't expect them to understand what I was going through. Their lives were going on as before; mine had changed. My perspectives and attitudes had a different focus than theirs. Many did not know what to say to me or how to relate. The ones who have stood by me and are still my friends, though few in number, have supported and enriched me.

I was bitter and resentful for a while about the

attitudes of some of the Christian young people in my church, but looking back I realize that God was using that situation to teach me whom to count on as real friends and to be content with who I am and my situation—instead of worrying about how others see me. God has let me know in a myriad of ways how important and valuable my son and I are to Him—that is what really matters!

I was prepared for the fact that when I decided to keep my child my dating life would certainly be restricted. I accepted that. I felt that time with my son was much more important than dates that would have little meaning to me now. I had learned that I did not need to have a boyfriend to be a complete and happy person. I had learned to love myself, and all I wanted to do was give to my son and be an integral part of my family. I concentrated on my son and my studies and left the rest to God. I knew that when it was best to bring someone into my life, God would do it in His time and in His way.

A year ago I met a guy at a church Christmas program. I had Eric with me at the time, and we had mutual friends—but I thought nothing would come of it. A few weeks later we were dating and have been ever since. He has come to love Eric as if he were his own. We are making plans to be married when I finish college and he gets settled in an occupation—that will probably be in two years or so. He wants to adopt Eric then. I couldn't be happier.

I am extremely proud of my son and where I am personally today in every area of my life. Nothing has been easy. I am not ashamed. I would not change my life if I could. This has been a blessed year. I have learned that God's timing and provisions are the best. I know that He is the One who gives the strength we need to get through our seasons of shadow.